CANCER OF THE BREAST

Brief guide on how to go about cancer of the breast

Dr. Maxwell Charlotte

Contents

CHAPTER ONE

INTRODUCTION

Breast cancer may be an illness within which cancerous (or malignant) cells develop uncontrollably within the breast tissue (usually in ducts - tubes that carry milk to the tit - or in the lobules - the milk manufacturing glands). It's the foremost common sort of cancer seen in ladies and also the leading reason behind death, in line with CSID.ro.

TYPES OF CARCINOMA

Breast cancer is usually classified into 2 types: non-invasive and invasive.

Non-invasive carcinoma or in place cancer carcinoma is found within the breasts of the breast. It can't be detected at the touching of the breast, however in an exceedingly X ray.

Invasive carcinoma extends on the far side the breast. the foremost common sort of carcinoma is invasive ductal carcinoma, that develops within the cells of the ducts.

Other kinds of carcinoma embrace invasive lobe breast cancer, inflammatory carcinoma and Paget's breast illness. sadly, invasive willcer|carcinoma} can unfold to alternative areas of the body.

More ladies are diagnosed with carcinoma than the other cancer, besides carcinoma. This year, associate degree calculable 268,600 ladies within the US are diagnosed with invasive carcinoma, and 62,930 ladies are diagnosed with in place carcinoma. Associate degree calculable a pair of,670 men within the us are diagnosed with carcinoma.

It is calculable that forty two,260 deaths (41,760 ladies and five hundred men) from carcinoma can occur this year.

The five-year survival rate tells you what p.c of individuals live a minimum of 5 years once the cancer is found. p.c means that what number out of a hundred. the common 5-year survival rate for girls with invasive carcinoma is ninetieth. the common 10-year survival rate is eighty three.

If the cancer is found solely within the breast, the 5-year survival rate of ladies with carcinoma is ninety nine. cardinal p.c (62%) of cases are diagnosed at this stage. If the cancer has unfold to the regional humor nodes, the 5-year survival rate is eighty fifth. If the cancer has unfolded to an overseas a part of the body, the 5-year survival rate is twenty seventh.

About 6 June 1944 of ladies have pathological process cancer once they are 1st diagnosed with carcinoma. Though the cancer is **found** at a additional advanced stage, new treatments facilitate many folks with carcinoma maintain an honest quality of life, a minimum of for a few time.

It is necessary to notice that these statistics are averages, and every person's risk depends on several factors, as well as the scale of the tumour, the amount of humour nodes that contain cancer, and alternative options of the tumour that have an effect on how quickly a tumor can grow and the way well treatment works. this implies that it is tough to estimate every person's probability of survival.

Breast cancer is that the second commonest reason behind death from cancer in ladies within the us, once carcinoma. However, since 1989, the amount of ladies UN agency has died of carcinoma has steady shriveled due to early detection and treatment enhancements.

Currently, there are quite three million ladies UN agencies are diagnosed with carcinoma within the us.

It is necessary to recollect that statistics on the survival rates for individuals with carcinoma are associate degree estimate. The estimate comes from annual information supported the amount of individuals with this cancer within the us. Also, consultants live the survival statistics each five years. therefore the estimate might not show the results of higher designation or treatment obtainable for fewer than five years. speak along with your doctor if you've got any questions about this info. Learn additional regarding understanding statistics.

CAUSES AND RISK FACTORS IN CARCINOMA

An exact reason behind this kind of cancer is unknown. Studies show that older age and feminine hormones play a crucial role within the development of this kind of cancer. it's common in ladies over fifty years more matured.

It's arduous to inform why some ladies will develop carcinoma et al. don't. There are risk factors that you'll amendment, however some ahead of whom you'll not do something.

• Age - eight out of ten ladies will have carcinoma once their fiftieth birthday.

• case history - if there are family-related cases, relatives of grade one and 2, the danger of developing this kind of cancer is incredibly high.

• Previous carcinoma or designation - if you've got antecedently had breast cancer or non-invasive neoplastic cell changes within the duct gland ducts, or sure kinds of nodules might increase the danger of developing cancer.

• Breast density - ladies UN agency have additional dense breast tissue might have the next risk of developing this illness.

• 1st menstruum at associate degree early age (less than twelve years old)

• actinotherapy for breasts or chest

• steroid hormone treatments

• Older age initially childbearing

• Overweight and avoirdupois

• Diet wealthy in fat

• Alcohol consumption

This section explains the kinds of treatments that are the quality of look after early-stage and domestically advanced carcinoma. "Standard of care" means that the simplest treatments identified. once creating treatment set up choices, you're inspired to contemplate clinical trials as associate degree choice. A trial may be a analysis study that tests a brand new approach to treatment. Doctors need to be told whether or not the new treatment is safe, effective, and presumably higher than the quality treatment. Clinical trials will take a look at a brand new drug and the way usually it ought to lean, a brand new combination of normal treatments, or new doses of normal medicine or alternative treatments. Some clinical trials additionally take a look at giving less treatment than what's sometimes done as normal of care. Clinical trials are associate degree choice to contemplate for treatment and look after all stages of cancer. Your doctor will assist you contemplate all of your treatment choices. to be told additional regarding clinical trials, see the regarding Clinical Trials and Latest analysis sections.

CHAPTER TWO

In cancer care, doctors specializing in numerous areas of cancer treatment—such as surgery, radiation medical specialty, and medical oncology—work along to make a patient's overall treatment set up that mixes differing types of treatments. this can be referred to as a multidisciplinary team. Cancer care groups embrace a range of alternative health care professionals, like doctor assistants, medical specialty nurses, social employees, pharmacists, counselors, nutritionists, and others. For individuals older than sixty five, a geriatric specialist or specialist may additionally be concerned in care. raise the doctor accountable of your treatment that health care professionals are a part of your treatment team and what they are doing. this may amendment over time as your health care wants change.

A treatment set up may be a outline of your cancer and also the planned cancer treatment. it's meant to grant basic info regarding your medical record to any doctors UN agency can look after you throughout your lifespan. Before treatment begins, raise your doctor for a duplicate of your treatment set up. you'll additionally give your doctor with a duplicate of the ASCO Treatment set up type to fill out.

The biology and behavior of carcinoma affects the treatment set up. Some tumors are smaller however grow quickly, whereas others are larger and grow slowly. Treatment choices and suggestions are terribly customized and rely upon many factors, including:

• The tumor's subtype, as well as secretion receptor standing (ER, PR) and HER2 standing (see Introduction)

• The stage of the tumour

• Genomic markers, like Oncotype DX™ and MammaPrint™ (if appropriate) (See Diagnosis)

• The patient's age, general health, biological time standing, and preferences

• The presence of identified mutations in hereditary carcinoma genes, like BRCA1 or BRCA2

Even though the carcinoma care team can specifically tailor the treatment for every patient and also the breast cancer, there are some general steps for treating early-stage and domestically advanced carcinoma.

For each DCIS and early-stage invasive carcinoma, doctors usually suggest surgery to get rid of the tumour. to create certain that the whole tumour is removed, the doc also will take away atiny low space of healthy tissue round the tumour, referred to as a margin. though the goal of surgery is to get rid of all of the visible cancer, microscopic cells is left behind, either within the breast or elsewhere. In some things, this implies that another surgery might be required to get rid of remaining cancer cells.

For larger cancers, or those who are growing additional quickly, doctors might suggest general treatment with therapy or secretion therapy before surgery, referred to as neoadjuvant medical aid. There is also many edges to having alternative treatments before surgery:

• ladies UN agency might have required a excision may have breast-conserving surgery (lumpectomy) if the tumour shrinks before surgery.

• Surgery is also easier to perform as a result of the tumour is smaller.

• Your doctor might decide if certain treatments work well for the cancer.

• you'll even be able to strive a brand new treatment through a trial.

After surgery, subsequent step in managing early-stage carcinoma is to lower the danger of return and to urge eliminate any remaining cancer cells. These cancer cells are undetectable however are believed to be liable for a cancer return as they will grow over time. Treatment given once surgery is named adjuvant medical aid. Adjuvant therapies might embrace radiotherapy, therapy, targeted medical aid, and/or secretion medical aid (see below for additional info on every of those treatments).

Whether adjuvant medical aid is required depends on the possibility that any cancer cells stay within the breast or the body and also the chance that a selected treatment can work to treat the cancer. though adjuvant medical aid lowers the danger of return, it doesn't fully get eliminate the danger.

Along with staging, alternative tools will facilitate estimate prognosis and assist you and your doctor build choices regarding adjuvant medical aid. This includes tests that may predict the danger of return by testing your tumour tissue (such as Oncotype Dx™ or MammaPrint™; see Diagnosis). Such tests may additionally facilitate your doctor higher perceive the risks from the cancer and whether or not therapy can help scale back those risks.

When surgery to get rid of the cancer isn't attainable, it's referred to as inoperable. The doctor can then suggest treating the cancer in alternative ways that. therapy, targeted medical aid, radiotherapy, and/or secretion medical aid is also given to shrink the cancer.

For perennial cancer, treatment choices rely upon however the cancer was 1st treated and also the characteristics of the cancer mentioned higher than, such as ER, PR, and HER2.

Descriptions of the common kinds of treatments used for early-stage and domestically advanced carcinoma are listed below. Your care set up additionally includes treatment for symptoms and facet effects, a crucial a part of cancer care. Take time to be told about all of your treatment choices and take care to raise questions about things that are unclear. speak along with your doctor regarding the goals of every treatment and what you'll expect whereas receiving the treatment. it's additionally necessary to examine along with your insurance company before any treatment begins to create certain it is coated.

People older than sixty five might have the benefit of having a geriatric assessment before coming up with treatment. decide what a geriatric assessment involves.

Learn additional regarding creating treatment choices.

Surgery is that the removal of the tumour and a few close healthy tissue throughout associate degree operation. Surgery is additionally wont to examine the close axillary humour nodes, that are underneath the arm. A surgical specialist may be a doctor UN agency makes a speciality of treating cancer with surgery. Learn additional regarding the fundamentals of cancer surgery.

Generally, the smaller the tumour, the additional surgical choices a patient has. the kinds of surgery embrace the following:

• extirpation. this can be the removal of the tumour and atiny low, cancer-free margin of healthy tissue round the tumour. Most of the breast remains. For invasive cancer, radiotherapy to the remaining breast tissue is usually suggested once surgery. For DCIS, radiotherapy once surgery is also associate degree choice reckoning on the patient and also the tumour. A extirpation may additionally be referred to as breast-conserving surgery, a partial excision, quadrantectomy, or a segmental excision.

• excision. this can be the surgical removal of the whole breast. There are many kinds of mastectomies. speak along with your doctor regarding whether or not the skin is preserved, referred to as a skin-sparing excision, or the tit, referred to as a complete skin-sparing excision.

CHAPTER THREE

Cancer cells is found within the axillary humour nodes in some cancers. it's necessary to search out out whether or not any of the humour nodes close to the breast contain cancer. This info is employed to see treatment and prognosis.

• watcher node diagnostic assay. in an exceedingly watcher node diagnostic assay, the doc finds and removes atiny low variety of humour nodes from underneath the arm that receive lymph drain from the breast. This procedure helps avoid removing multiple nodes with associate degree axillary humour node dissection (see below) for patients whose watcher lymph nodes are principally freed from cancer. The smaller node procedure helps lower the danger of many attainable facet effects. Those facet effects embrace swelling of the arm referred to as oedema, the danger of symptom, likewise as arm movement and range-of-motion issues with the shoulder, that are long-lived problems that may severely have an effect on a person's quality of life.

The diagnostician then examines these humour nodes for cancer cells. to search out the watcher node, the doc sometimes injects a dye and/or a hot tracer behind or round the tit. The injection, which may cause some discomfort, lasts regarding fifteen seconds. The dye or tracer travels to the humour nodes, inbound at the watcher node 1st. The doc will notice the node once it turns color if the dye is employed or offers off radiation if the tracer is used.

If the watcher node is cancer-free, analysis has shown that it's doubtless that the remaining humour nodes also will be freed from cancer. this implies that no additional humour nodes got to be removed. If only one or a pair of watcher humour nodes have cancer and you intend to own a extirpation and radiotherapy to the whole breast, associate degree axillary node dissection might not be not required. decide additional regarding   ASCO's recommendations for watcher node diagnostic assay.

• Axillary node dissection. In associate degree axillary node dissection, the doc removes several humour nodes from underneath the arm. These are then examined by a diagnostician for cancer cells. the particular variety of humour nodes removed varies from person to person. associate degree axillary node dissection might not be required for all ladies with early-stage carcinoma with little amounts of cancer within the watcher humour nodes. ladies having a extirpation and radiotherapy UN agency have a smaller tumour and no quite a pair of watcher nodes with cancer might avoid a full axillary humour node dissection. This helps scale back the danger of facet effects and doesn't decrease survival. If cancer is found within the watcher node, whether or not additional surgery is required to get rid of more humour nodes depends on the particular scenario.

Most people with invasive carcinoma can have either a watcher node diagnostic assay or an axillary lymph node dissection. However, these procedures is also elective for a few patients older than sixty five. this relies on however giant the humour nodes are, the tumor's stage, and also the person's overall health.

A watcher node diagnostic assay alone might not be done if there's obvious proof of cancer within the humour nodes before any surgery. during this scenario, a full axillary node dissection is most well-liked.

Normally, the humour nodes don't seem to be evaluated for patients with DCIS and no invasive cancer, since the danger of unfold is incredibly low. However, the doc might contemplate a watcher node diagnostic assay for patients diagnosed with DCIS UN agency prefer to have or want a excision. If some invasive cancer is found with DCIS throughout the excision, that happens sometimes, the humour nodes can then got to be evaluated. Once the breast tissue has been removed with a excision, it's harder to search out the watcher humour nodes since it is not as obvious wherever to inject the dye.

RECONSTRUCTIVE (PLASTIC) SURGERY

Women UN agency have a excision might want to contemplate breast reconstruction. this can be surgery to re-create a breast victimisation either tissue taken from another a part of the body or artificial implants. Reconstruction is sometimes performed by a sawbones. a lady is also able to have reconstruction at identical time because the excision, referred to as immediate reconstruction. She may additionally have it at some purpose within the future, referred to as delayed reconstruction.

For patients having a extirpation, reconstruction is also done at identical time to enhance the planning of the breast and to match the breasts. this can be referred to as oncoplastic surgery. several breast surgeons will do that while not the assistance of a sawbones. Surgery on the healthy breast may additionally be recommended so each breasts have an identical look.

The techniques mentioned below are usually wont to form a brand new breast.

Implants. A implant uses saline-filled or silicone polymer gel-filled forms to reshape the breast. the surface of a saline-filled implant is created from silicone polymer, and it's full of sterile saline, that is salt water. silicone polymer gel-filled implants are full of silicone rather than saline. They were thought to cause animal tissue disorders, however clear proof of this has not been found. Before having permanent implants, a lady might briefly have a tissue expander placed that may produce the right sized pocket for the implant. speak along with your doctor regarding the advantages and risks of silicone polymer versus saline implants. The period of an implant depends on the girl. However, some ladies ne'er got to have them replaced. alternative necessary factors to contemplate once selecting implants include:

• Saline implants generally "ripple" at the highest or shift with time, however many ladies don't notice it pestiferous enough to exchange.

• Saline implants tend to feel totally different than silicone polymer implants. they're usually firmer to the bit than silicone polymer implants.

There is issues with breast implants. Some ladies have issues with the form or look. and also the implants will rupture or break, cause pain and connective tissue round the implant, or get infected. they need additionally been seldom joined to alternative kinds of cancer. though these issues are terribly uncommon, speak along with your doctor regarding the risks.

Tissue flap procedures. These techniques use muscle and tissue from elsewhere within the body to reshape the breast. Tissue flap surgery is also finished a "pedicle flap," which suggests tissue from the rear or belly is affected to the chest while not cutting the blood vessels. A "free flap" means that the blood vessels are cut and also the doc must attach the affected tissue to new blood vessels within the chest. There are many flap procedures:

- cross musculus abdominis muscle (TRAM) flap. This technique, which may be done as a peduncle flap or free flap, uses muscle and tissue from the lower abdomen wall.

- Latissimus dorsi flap. This peduncle flap technique uses muscle and tissue from the higher back.

- Deep inferior artery perforator (DIEP) flap. The DIEP free flap takes tissue from the abdomen and also the doc attaches the blood vessels to the chest wall.

- skeletal muscle free flap. The skeletal muscle free flap uses tissue and muscle from the buttocks to make the breast, {and the|and therefore the|and additionally the} doc also attaches the blood vessels.

Because blood vessels are involved flap procedures, these methods are sometimes not suggested for a lady with a history of {diabetes|polygenic disorder|polygenic illness} or animal tissue or vascular disease, or for a lady UN agency smokes, because the risk of issues throughout and once surgery is far higher.

The DIEP and skeletal muscle free flap procedures are longer procedures and also the recovery time is longer. However, the looks of the breast is also most well-liked, particularly once radiotherapy is a component of the treatment set up.

Talk along with your doctor for additional info regarding

reconstruction choices. once considering a sawbones, select a doctor UN agency has expertise with a range of rehabilitative surgeries, as well as implants and flap procedures, and might discuss the execs and cons of every procedure.

EXTERNAL BREAST FORMS (PROSTHESES)

An external breast restorative or artificial breast type provides associate degree choice for girls UN agency attempt to delay or not have surgical operation. These is fabricated from silicone polymer or soft material, and match into a excision bandeau. Breast prostheses is created to produce an honest match and natural look for every girl.

To summarize, surgical procedure choices embrace the following:

• Removal of cancer within the breast: extirpation or partial excision, usually followed by radiotherapy if the cancer is invasive. radiotherapy might or might not be used if it's DCIS. A excision may additionally be suggested, with or while not immediate reconstruction.

• node evaluation: watcher lymph node diagnostic assay and/or axillary lymph node dissection.

Women are inspired to speak with their doctors regarding that surgical choice is true for them. Also, speak along with your health care team regarding the attainable facet effects from the particular surgery you may have.

More aggressive surgery, like a excision, isn't forever higher and will cause additional complications. the mix of extirpation and radiotherapy includes a slightly higher risk of the cancer returning within the same breast or the encompassing space. However, the long-run survival of ladies who select extirpation is precisely identical as people who have a excision. Even with a excision, not all breast tissue is removed and there's still an opportunity of return.

Women with a awfully high risk of developing a brand new cancer within the alternative breast might contemplate a bilateral excision, which means each breasts are removed. This includes women with BRCA1 or BRCA2 cistron mutations and girls with cancer in each breasts. for girls not at terribly high risk of developing a brand new cancer within the future, having a healthy breast removed in an exceedingly bilateral excision neither prevents cancer return nor improves a woman's survival. though the danger of obtaining a brand new cancer in this breast are down, surgery to get rid of the opposite breast doesn't scale back the danger of the first cancer returning. And additional intensive surgery is also joined with a bigger risk of issues.

CHAPTER FOUR

RADIATION MEDICAL AID

Radiation therapy is that the use of high-energy x-rays or alternative particles to destroy cancer cells. A doctor UN agency makes a speciality of giving radiotherapy to treat cancer is named a radiation specialist. There are many differing types of radiotherapy:

• External-beam radiotherapy. this can be the foremost common sort of radiation treatment and is given from a machine outside the body.

• Intra-operative radiotherapy. this can be once radiation treatment is given employing a probe within the surgery.

- Brachytherapy. this kind of radiotherapy is given by putting hot sources into the tumour.

Although the analysis results are encouraging, intra-operative radiotherapy and brachytherapy don't seem to be wide used. wherever obtainable, they'll be choices for patient with atiny low tumour that has not unfold to the humour nodes. Learn additional regarding the fundamentals of radiotherapy.

A radiotherapy programme, or schedule (see below), sometimes consists of a selected variety of treatments given over a collection amount of your time. radiotherapy usually helps lower the danger of return within the breast. In fact, with fashionable surgery and radiotherapy, return rates within the breast are currently but five-hitter in the ten years once treatment, and survival is that the same with extirpation or excision. If there's cancer within the humour nodes underneath the arm, radiotherapy may additionally lean to identical facet of the neck or underarm close to the breast or chest wall.

Radiation therapy is also given once or before surgery:

• Adjuvant radiotherapy is given once surgery. most ordinarily, it's given once a extirpation, and generally, therapy. Patients UN agency have a excision might not want radiotherapy, reckoning on the options of the tumour. radiotherapy is also suggested once excision if you've got a bigger tumour, cancer within the humour nodes, cancer cells outside of the capsule of the node, or cancer that has full-grown into the skin or chest wall, likewise as for alternative reasons.

• Neoadjuvant radiotherapy is radiation therapy given before surgery to shrink an outsized tumour, that makes it easier to get rid of. This approach is unusual and is simply thought of once a tumour can't be removed with surgery.

Radiation therapy will cause facet effects, as well as fatigue, swelling of the breast, redness and/or skin discoloration or physiological condition, and pain or burning within the skin wherever the radiation was directed, generally with blistering or peeling. Your doctor will suggest topical medication to use to the skin to treat a number of these facet effects.

Very seldom, atiny low quantity of the respiratory organ is littered with the radiotherapy, inflicting redness, a radiation-related swelling of the respiratory organ tissue. This risk depends on the scale of the world that received radiotherapy, and this tends to heal with time.

In the past, with older instrumentation and radiotherapy techniques, ladies UN agency received treatment for carcinoma on the left facet of the body had atiny low increase within the long-run risk of cardiovascular disease. fashionable techniques are currently able to spare the overwhelming majority of the center from the results of radiotherapy.

Many types of radiotherapy is also obtainable to you with totally different schedules (see below). speak along with your doctor regarding the benefits and drawbacks of every choice.

RADIATION THERAPY SCHEDULE

Radiation therapy is sometimes given daily for a collection variety of weeks.

• once a extirpation. radiotherapy once a extirpation is external-beam radiation therapy given Mon through Fri for three to four weeks if the cancer isn't within the humour nodes. If the cancer is within the humour nodes, radiotherapy is given for five to six weeks. This usually starts with radiotherapy to the total breast, followed by a additional targeted treatment to wherever the tumour was settled within the breast for the remaining treatments.

This targeted a part of the treatment, referred to as a lift, is normal for girls with invasive carcinoma to scale back the danger of a return within the breast. ladies with DCIS may additionally receive the boost. for girls with a coffee risk of return, the boost is also elective. it's necessary to debate this treatment approach along with your doctor.

• once a excision. For people who want radiotherapy once a excision, it's sometimes given 5 days per week for five to six weeks. radiotherapy is given before or once surgical operation.

Even shorter schedules are studied and are in use in some centers, as well as accelerated partial breast radiotherapy (see below) for five days.

These shorter schedules might not be choices for girls UN agency want radiotherapy once a excision or radiotherapy to their humour nodes. Also, longer schedules of radiotherapy is also required for a few ladies with terribly giant breasts. additional analysis is being done to search out out whether or not younger patients or people who want radiotherapy once therapy is also able to have these shorter radiation therapy schedules.

• Partial breast irradiation. Partial breast irradiation (PBI) is radiotherapy that's given on to the tumour space rather than the whole breast. it's additional common once a extirpation. Targeting radiation on to the tumour space sometimes shortens the quantity of your time that patients got to receive radiotherapy. However, just some patients is also able to have PBI. though early results are promising, PBI remains being studied. it's the topic of an outsized, nationwide trial, and also the results on the protection and effectiveness compared with normal radiotherapy don't seem to be however prepared. This study can facilitate decide that patients are the foremost doubtless to profit from PBI.

PBI is finished normal external-beam radiotherapy that's targeted on the world wherever tumour was removed and not on the whole breast. PBI may additionally be finished brachytherapy by victimisation plastic catheters or a metal wand placed briefly within the breast. Breast brachytherapy will involve short treatment times, starting from one dose to 1 week. It may lean as one dose within the surgery in real time once the tumour is removed. These styles of targeted radiotherapy are presently used just for patients with a smaller, less-aggressive, and humour node-negative tumour.

• Intensity-modulated radiotherapy. Intensity-modulated radiotherapy (IMRT) may be a additional advanced thanks to provide external-beam radiation therapy to the breast. The intensity of the radiation directed at the breast is varied to higher target the tumour, spreading the radiation additional equally throughout the breast. the utilization of IMRT lessens the radiation dose and will decrease attainable harm to close organs, like the center and respiratory organ, and also the risks of some immediate facet effects, like peeling of the skin throughout treatment. this may be particularly necessary for girls with medium to giant breasts UN agency have the next risk of facet effects, like peeling and burns, compared with ladies with smaller breasts. IMRT may additionally facilitate to reduce the long-run effects on the breast tissue, like hardness, swelling, or discoloration, that were common with older radiation techniques.

IMRT isn't suggested for everybody. speak along with your radiation specialist to be told additional. Special insurance approval may additionally be required for coverage for IMRT. it's necessary to examine along with your insurance company before any treatment begins to create certain it is coated.

• nucleon medical aid. normal radiotherapy for carcinoma uses x-rays, additionally referred to as gauge boson medical aid, to kill cancer cells. nucleon therapy may be a sort of external-beam radiotherapy that uses protons instead of x-rays. At high energy, protons will destroy cancer cells. Protons have totally different physical properties that will enable the radiotherapy to be additional targeted than gauge boson therapy and probably scale back the radiation dose. The medical aid may additionally scale back the quantity of radiation that goes close to the center. Researchers are finding out the advantages of nucleon medical aid versus gauge boson therapy in an exceedingly national trial. Currently, nucleon medical aid is associate degree experimental treatment and will not be wide obtainable.

Adjuvant radiotherapy considerations for older patients and/or those with atiny low tumour

Recent analysis studies have checked out the chance of avoiding radiotherapy for girls age seventy or older with associate degree ER-positive, early-stage tumour (see Introduction), or for those ladies with atiny low tumour. Overall, these studies show that radiotherapy reduces the danger of carcinoma return within the same breast, compared with no radiotherapy. However, radiotherapy doesn't lengthen women's lives.

Guidelines from the National Comprehensive Cancer Network (NCCN) still suggest radiotherapy because the normal choice once extirpation. However, they note that girls with special things or a low-risk tumour may moderately select to not have radiotherapy and use solely general therapy (see below) once extirpation. This includes ladies age seventy or older and people with alternative medical conditions that might limit lifespan inside five years. people that select this selection should be caning to just accept a modest increase within the risk that the cancer will come in the breast.

THERAPIES VICTIMISATION MEDICATION

Systemic medical aid is that the use of medication to destroy cancer cells. this kind of medication is given through the blood to achieve cancer cells throughout the body. general therapies are usually prescribed by a medical specialist, a doctor UN agency makes a speciality of treating cancer with medication.

Common ways that to grant general therapies embrace associate degree endovenous (IV) tube placed into a vein employing a needle, associate degree injection into a muscle or underneath the skin, or in an exceedingly pill or capsule that's enclosed (orally).

The types of general therapies used for carcinoma include:

• therapy

• secretion medical aid

• Targeted medical aid

• therapy

Each of those therapies are mentioned below in additional detail. an individual might receive only 1 sort of general medical aid at a time or a mixture of systemic therapies given at identical time. they will even be given as a part of a treatment set up that features surgery and/or radiotherapy.

The medications wont to treat cancer are regularly being evaluated. Talking along with your doctor is usually the simplest thanks to find out about the medications prescribed for you, their purpose, and their potential facet effects. it's additionally necessary to let your doctor apprehend if you're taking any prescription or over-the-counter medications or supplements. Herbs, supplements, and alternative medicine will move with cancer medications. Learn additional regarding your prescriptions by victimisation searchable drug databases.

CHAPTER FIVE

CHEMOTHERAPY

Chemotherapy is that the use of medicine to destroy cancer cells, sometimes by ending the cancer cells' ability to grow and divide. it should lean before surgery to shrink an outsized tumour, build surgery easier, and scale back the danger of return, referred to as neoadjuvant therapy. it should even be given once surgery to scale back the danger of return, referred to as adjuvant therapy.

A therapy programme, or schedule, sometimes consists of a mixture of medicine given in an exceedingly specific variety of cycles over a collection amount of your time. therapy is also given on many various schedules reckoning on what worked best in clinical trials for that specific sort of programme. it should lean once per week, once each a pair of weeks (also referred to as dose-dense), once each three weeks, or perhaps once each four weeks. There are many varieties of therapy wont to treat carcinoma. Common medicine include:

• Capecitabine (Xeloda)

• Carboplatin (available as a generic drug)

• Cisplatin (available as a generic drug)

• Cyclophosphamide (available as a generic drug)

• Docetaxel (Taxotere)

• antibiotic drug (available as a generic drug)

- Pegylated liposomal antibiotic drug (Doxil)

- Epirubicin (Ellence)

- Eribulin (Halaven)

- antimetabolite (5-FU, Efudex)

- Gemcitabine (Gemzar)

- Ixabepilone (Ixempra)

- amethopterin (Rheumatrex, Trexall)

- Paclitaxel (Taxol)

- Protein-bound paclitaxel (Abraxane)

- Vinorelbine (Navelbine)

A patient might receive one drug at a time or a mixture of various medicine given at identical time. analysis has shown that combos of sure medicine are generally more practical than single drugs for adjuvant treatment. the subsequent drugs or combos of medicine is also used as adjuvant medical aid for early-stage and domestically advanced breast cancer:

- AC (doxorubicin and cyclophosphamide)

- EU (epirubicin, cyclophosphamide)

- AC or EU (epirubicin and cyclophosphamide) followed by T (doxorubicin and cyclophosphamide, followed by paclitaxel or docetaxel, or the reverse)

- CAF (cyclophosphamide, antibiotic drug, and 5-FU)

- CEF (cyclophosphamide, epirubicin, and 5-FU)

- CMF (cyclophosphamide, amethopterin, and 5-FU)

- TAC (docetaxel, antibiotic drug, and cyclophosphamide)

- TC (docetaxel and cyclophosphamide)

Therapies that focus on the HER2 receptor is also given with therapy for HER2-positive carcinoma (see Targeted medical aid, below). associate degree example is that the protein trastuzumab. Combination regimens for early-stage HER2-positive carcinoma might include:

- AC-TH (doxorubicin, cyclophosphamide, paclitaxel, trastuzumab)

- AC-THP (doxorubicin, cyclophosphamide, paclitaxel, trastuzumab, pertuzumab)

- TCHP (docetaxel, carboplatin, trastuzumab, pertuzumab)

- TCH (docetaxel, carboplatin, trastuzumab)

- TH (paclitaxel, trastuzumab)

The facet effects of therapy rely upon the individual, the drug(s) used, and also the schedule and dose used. These facet effects will embrace fatigue, risk of infection, nausea and forcing out, hair loss, loss of appetence, diarrhea, constipation, early change of life, weight gain, and chemo-brain. These facet effects will usually be terribly with success prevented or managed throughout treatment with accessory medications, and that they sometimes escape once treatment is finished. Rarely, long-run facet effects might occur, like heart harm, nerve harm, or secondary cancers like leukaemia and malignant neoplastic disease. several patients feel well throughout therapy and are actively taking care of their families, working, and workout throughout treatment, though every person's expertise is totally different. speak along with your health care team regarding the attainable facet effects of your specific therapy set up.

Learn additional regarding the fundamentals of therapy.

Hormonal medical aid

Hormonal medical aid, additionally referred to as endocrine medical aid, is an efficient treatment for many tumors that take a look at positive for either steroid hormone or progestogen receptors (called ER-positive or PR-positive; see Introduction). this kind of tumour uses hormones to fuel its growth. interference the hormones will facilitate stop a cancer return and death from carcinoma once used either by itself or once therapy.

Hormonal medical aid is also given before surgery to shrink a tumour, build surgery easier, and lower the danger of return. this can be referred to as neoadjuvant secretion medical aid. it should even be given once surgery to scale back the danger of return. this can be referred to as adjuvant secretion medical aid.

TYPES OF SECRETION MEDICAL AID
• antagonist. antagonist may be a drug that blocks steroid hormone from binding to carcinoma cells. it's effective for lowering the

danger of return within the breast that had cancer, the danger of developing cancer within the alternative breast, and also the risk of distant return. antagonist works well in ladies UN agency are through change of life and people who haven't.

Tamoxifen may be a pill that's taken daily orally. it's necessary to debate the other medications or supplements you're taking along with your doctor, as there are some that will interfere with antagonist. Common facet effects of antagonist embrace hot flashes likewise as canal status, discharge or injury. terribly rare risks embrace a cancer of the liner of the womb, cataracts, and blood clots. However, antagonist might improve bone health and cholesterin levels.

• Aromatase inhibitors (AIs). AIs decrease the quantity of steroid hormone created in tissues aside from the ovaries in biological time ladies by interference the aromatase accelerator. This accelerator changes weak male hormones referred to as androgens into steroid hormone once the ovaries have stopped creating estrogen throughout change of life. These medicine embrace anastrozole (Arimidex), exemestane (Aromasin), and letrozole (Femara). All of the AIs are pills taken daily orally. solely ladies UN agency have undergone change of life or who have had medicines to prevent the ovaries from creating steroid hormone (see female internal reproductive organ suppression, below) will take AIs. Treatment with AIs, either because the 1st secretion medical aid taken or once treatment with antagonist, is also more practical than taking solely antagonist to scale back the danger of return in post-menopausal ladies.

The facet effects of AIs might embrace muscle and joint pain, hot flashes, canal status, associate degree augmented risk of pathology and broken bones, and augmented cholesterin levels. analysis shows that each one AIs work equally well and have similar facet effects. However, ladies UN agency have undesirable facet effects whereas taking associate degree AI might have fewer side effects with another AI for unclear reasons.

Women UN agency haven't undergone change of life mustn't take AIs, as they are doing not block the results of steroid hormone created by the ovaries. Often, doctors can monitor blood steroid hormone levels in ladies whose expelling cycles have recently stopped, or those whose periods stop with therapy to take care that the ovaries aren't any longer manufacturing steroid hormone.

• female internal reproductive organ suppression. female internal reproductive organ suppression is that the use of medicine or surgery to prevent the ovaries from manufacturing steroid hormone. it should be employed in addition to a different sort of secretion medical aid for girls UN agency haven't been through change of life. There are a pair of ways used for female internal reproductive organ suppression:

o gonadotrophin or luteinizing cathartic hormone (GnRH or LHRH) medicine stop the ovaries from creating steroid hormone, inflicting temporary change of life. Goserelin (Zoladex) and leuprolide (Eligard, Lupron) are kinds of these medicine. they're given by injection and stop the ovaries from creating steroid hormone for one to three months. the results of GnRH medicine escape if treatment is stopped.

o Surgery to get rid of the ovaries, that additionally stops steroid hormone production. whereas this can be permanent, it is an honest choice for girls UN agency are done having youngsters, particularly since the price is often lower over the future.

Hormonal medical aid for girls once change of life

Women UN agency have undergone change of life and are prescribed secretion medical aid have many options:

• antagonist for five to ten years

• associate degree AI for five to ten years

• antagonist for five years, followed by associate degree AI for up to five years. this may be a complete of ten years of secretion medical aid.

• antagonist for two to three years, followed by a pair of to eight years of associate degree AI for a complete of five to ten years of secretion medical aid.

In general, ladies with stage I cancer ought to expect to require secretion medical aid for five years. ladies with stage II or III cancer might expect to require it for up to ten years.

Hormonal medical aid for biological time ladies

As noted higher than, biological time ladies mustn't take solely AIs, as they'll not work. choices for adjuvant secretion medical aid for biological time ladies embrace the following:

• antagonist for five years. Then, treatment relies on whether or not or not they need undergone change of life in those five years.

o If a lady has not undergone change of life once the primary five years of treatment, she will be able to continue antagonist for one more five years, for a complete of ten years of antagonist.

o If a lady goes through change of life throughout the primary five years of treatment, she will be able to continue antagonist for a further 5 years or switch to an AI for five additional years. this may be a complete of ten years of secretion medical aid. solely ladies UN agency are clearly biological time ought to contemplate taking associate degree AI.

• female internal reproductive organ suppression for five years beside extra secretion medical aid, like {tamoxifen|estrogen associate degreetagonist|antagonist} or an

AI, is also suggested within the following things, reckoning on a woman's age and risk of recurrence:

o for girls UN agency are diagnosed with carcinoma at a awfully young age.

o for girls UN agency have a high risk of cancer return.

o for girls with stage II or stage III cancer once therapy is additionally suggested.

o for girls with stage I or stage II cancer with the next risk of return UN agency might contemplate additionally having therapy.

o for girls UN agency cannot take antagonist for alternative health reasons, like having a history of blood clots.

- female internal reproductive organ suppression isn't suggested additionally to a different sort of secretion medical aid within the following situations:

o for girls with cancer that's not terribly doubtless to recur.

o for girls with stage I cancer once therapy has not been suggested.

This info relies on ASCO recommendations for adjuvant endocrine medical aid for girls with secretion receptor-positive carcinoma. Please note this link takes you to a different ASCO web site.

THE END